AF492912

Table of Contents

INTRODUCTION

Shibboleth Diet is more than just a weight loss diet it's a lifestyle you could live with in the long term. The Shibboleth Diet is a behavior modification program that helps each person on a day-to-day basis. Every day, as we strive to better ourselves, this diet makes it easier to follow through. First, your aim should be clear. If you have an obesity problem, for example, and you want to shed some excess pounds then this diet can help you out from this problem. The best part of this diet is that the shibboleth diet is an easy and simple diet to follow.

Anyone can follow this diet program easily because the shibboleth diet sets a path according to your lifestyle no matter if you are vegetarian, a workout enthusiast, or have a busy lifestyle. These things don't matter in this diet program. As mentioned, this diet is combining lifestyle and behavior modifications. You can eat whatever you like to eat as long as it's healthy and following the diet. Understanding the lifestyle is crucial for success with the Shibboleth Diet because thoughts lead to action and action leads to habits. Say goodbye to junk food if you are following the Shibboleth Diet. There are many food recipes that you can eat during this diet program.

RECEPIES

Homemade Chorizo

Ingredients

1 clove garlic

3 teaspoons dried oregano

½ cup distilled white vinegar

½ cup crushed red pepper flakes

½ cup water

2 ½ pounds ground pork

Directions

Step 1

In a blender, combine garlic, oregano, vinegar, red pepper flakes, and water. Blend until smooth.

Step 2

In a bowl pour mixture over ground pork; cover and refrigerate all day. Pour off any water that accumulates. Refrigerate or freeze for future use.

Nutrition Facts Per Serving:

321.7 calories; protein 26.3g 53% DV; carbohydrates 5.5g 2% DV; fat 21.9g 34% DV; cholesterol 92mg 31% DV; sodium 74.7mg 3% DV.

Easy Chicken Taco Filling

Ingredients

2 breast half, bone and skin removed (blank)s skinless, boneless chicken breast halves

¼ onion, sliced

¼ green bell pepper, sliced

Directions

Step 1

Saute onion and bell pepper in a medium skillet until soft.

Step 2

Place chicken breasts on top of saute mixture and spray with cooking spray.

Step 3

Fry chicken with saute mixture until browned and cooked through, cutting or shredding chicken while it cooks.

Prime Rib

Ingredients

1 (10 pound) prime rib roast

6 cloves garlic, sliced

salt and ground black pepper to taste

½ cup Dijon mustard

Directions

Step 1

Preheat the oven to 500 degrees F (260 degrees C).

Step 2

Make slits all over the roast by pricking with a small knife. Insert slivers of sliced garlic. Season the roast with salt and pepper, then spread generously with mustard. Place on a rack in a roasting pan, and cover.

Step 3

Roast for 60 minutes in the preheated oven. Turn off oven. Leave oven closed, and do not peek for 90 minutes. The internal temperature of the meat should be at least

Nutrition Facts Per Serving:

443.4 calories; protein 46.5g 93% DV; carbohydrates 2.6g 1% DV; fat 25.7g 40% DV; cholesterol 132.5mg 44% DV; sodium 364.6mg 15% DV.

Kim's Prime Rib

Ingredients

5 pounds rib roast

¼ cup soy sauce

¼ cup Worcestershire sauce

½ teaspoon garlic powder

onion salt

1 tablespoon browning sauce

1 ½ cups water

Directions

Step 1

Preheat oven to 450 degrees F (230 degrees C).

Step 2

In a medium bowl, combine the soy sauce, Worcestershire sauce, garlic powder, onion salt, browning sauce and water. Place roast in a roasting pan ribs side down and poke deep holes in the roast with a knife. Pour the marinade over the roast. Using a baster, squirt marinade into the holes you created with the knife and over the entire roast a few times.

Step 3

Bake at 450 degrees F (230 degrees C) for about 1 hour. (Note: Bake for 40 to 45 minutes for a smaller roast so that it does not dry out.)

Step 4

Remove roast from oven and reduce temperature in the oven to 200 degrees F (95 degrees C).

Step 5

When oven has reached 200 degrees F (95 degrees C), return roast to oven and continue cooking for 18 to 22 minutes per pound, or until internal temperature reaches 145 degrees F (65 degrees C).

Nutrition Facts Per Serving:

614.2 calories; protein 50.8g 102% DV; carbohydrates 3.9g 1% DV; fat 42.3g 65% DV; cholesterol 162.7mg 54% DV; sodium 982.3mg 39% DV.

Rock Salt Roast Prime Rib

Ingredients

1 (4 pound) prime rib roast

2 cups prepared hot mustard

4 cups rock salt

1 cup cream

2 tablespoons prepared horseradish

Directions

Step 1

Preheat oven to 450 degrees F (230 degrees C). Line a roasting pan with aluminum foil.

Step 2

Liberally coat the roast with mustard, so that it is entirely covered. Put a thick layer of rock salt on the foil in the roasting pan, about the size of the bottom of the roast. Set the bottom of the roast on the salt, and press down to embed the salt into the mustard. Completely cover the remainder of the roast with rock salt, pressing it into the mustard. (A lot of salt will fall off into the pan, but that doesn't hurt anything).

Step 3

Bake uncovered, in preheated oven for 60 minutes, or until internal temperature reaches 145 degrees F (65 degrees C). Let stand 15 minutes. The roast will be encased in a 'shell'. Hit the shell sharply with the back of a knife, and it will crack open and start to fall off. Remove the shell, and place the roast on a cutting board. Slice, and serve with horseradish sauce.

Step 4

Horseradish sauce: In a small bowl, whip the cream until stiff peaks form. Fold in horseradish to taste.

Nutrition Facts Per Serving:

2020.2 calories; protein 80.3g 161% DV; carbohydrates 10.6g 4% DV; fat 183.8g 283% DV; cholesterol 420.2mg 140% DV; sodium 112558.4mg 4690% DV.

Best Prime Rib Roast

Ingredients

3 teaspoons grated fresh ginger root

⅓ cup orange marmalade

4 cloves garlic, minced

3 tablespoons soy sauce

2 tablespoons brown sugar

¼ teaspoon hot pepper sauce

1 tablespoon mustard powder

1 cup beer

1 (8 pound) prime rib roast

¼ cup olive oil

freshly ground black pepper

Directions

Step 1

Mix together the ginger, marmalade, garlic, soy sauce, brown sugar, hot sauce, and mustard. Stir in the beer. Prick holes all over the roast with a 2 pronged fork. Pour marinade over roast. Cover, and refrigerate for at least 2 hours, basting at least twice.

Step 2

Preheat oven to 400 degrees F (200 degrees C).

Step 3

Place roast on a rack in a roasting pan. Pour about 1 cup of marinade into the roasting pan, and discard remaining marinade. Pour olive oil over roast, and season with freshly ground black pepper. Insert a roasting thermometer into the middle of the roast, making sure that the thermometer does not touch any bone. Cover roasting pan with aluminum foil, and seal edges tightly around pan.

Step 4

Cook roast for 1 hour in the preheated oven. After the first hour, remove the aluminum foil. Baste, reduce heat to 325 degrees F (165 degrees C), and continue roasting for 1 more hour. The thermometer reading should be at least 140 degrees F (60 degrees C) for medium-rare, and 170 degrees F (76 degrees C) for well done. Remove roasting pan from oven, place aluminum foil over roast, and let rest for about 30 minutes before slicing.

Nutrition Facts Per Serving:

629.6 calories; protein 30.1g 60% DV; carbohydrates 9.9g 3% DV; fat 50.9g 78% DV; cholesterol 112.6mg 38% DV; sodium 319.7mg 13% DV.

LuvAnn's Guacamole

Ingredients

2 avocado, NS as to Florida or Californias avocados - peeled, pitted and diced

2 teaspoons salt, or to taste

1 large tomato, diced

1 onion, diced

2 peppers jalapeno peppers, chopped

½ tablespoon chopped fresh cilantro

2 tablespoons fresh lime juice

Directions

Step 1

In a medium bowl, mash the avocados and stir in salt to taste. Mix in the tomato, onion, jalapeno, cilantro and lime juice. Cover and chill in the refrigerator at least 30 minutes before serving.

Nutrition Facts Per Serving:

46 calories; protein 0.7g 1% DV; carbohydrates 3.5g 1% DV; fat 3.7g 6% DV; cholesterolmg; sodium 293.4mg 12% DV.

Easy Guacamole

Ingredients

2 avocado, NS as to Florida or Californias avocados

1 small onion, finely chopped

1 clove garlic, minced

1 ripe tomato, chopped

1 lime, juiced

salt and pepper to taste

Directions

Step 1

Peel and mash avocados in a medium serving bowl. Stir in onion, garlic, tomato, lime juice, salt and pepper. Season with remaining lime juice and salt and pepper to taste. Chill for half an hour to blend flavors.

Nutrition Facts Per Serving:

44.9 calories; protein 0.7g 1% DV; carbohydrates 3.4g 1% DV; fat 3.7g 6% DV; cholesterolmg; sodium 2.4mg.

Best Guacamole

Ingredients

2 avocado, NS as to Florida or Californias avocados

½ lemon, juiced

2 tablespoons chopped onion

½ teaspoon salt

2 tablespoons olive oil

Directions

Step 1

Cut the avocados into halves. Remove the seeds, and scoop out the pulp into a small bowl. Use a fork to mash the avocado. Stir in lemon juice, onion, salt, and olive oil. Cover the bowl, and refrigerate for 1 hour before serving.

Nutrition Facts Per Serving:

56.3 calories; protein 0.6g 1% DV; carbohydrates 2.6g 1% DV; fat 5.4g 8% DV; cholesterolmg; sodium 74.6mg 3% DV.

Traditional Mexican Guacamole

Ingredients

2 medium (blank)s avocados, peeled and pitted

1 cup chopped tomatoes

¼ cup chopped onion

¼ cup chopped cilantro

2 tablespoons lemon juice

1 jalapeno pepper, seeded and minced

1 pinch salt and ground black pepper to taste

Directions

Step 1

Mash avocados in a bowl until creamy.

Step 2

Mix tomatoes, onion, cilantro, lemon juice, and jalapeno pepper into mashed avocado until well combined; season with salt and black pepper.

Nutrition Facts Per Serving:

176.5 calories; protein 2.7g 5% DV; carbohydrates 12.2g 4% DV; fat 14.9g 23% DV; cholesterolmg; sodium 49.9mg 2% DV.

Insalata Caprese II

Ingredients

4 large ripe tomatoes, sliced 1/4 inch thick

1 pound fresh mozzarella cheese, sliced 1/4 inch thick

⅓ cup fresh basil leaves

3 tablespoons extra virgin olive oil

½ teaspoon fine sea salt to taste

1 pinch freshly ground black pepper to taste

Directions

Step 1

On a large platter, alternate and overlap the tomato slices, mozzarella cheese slices, and basil leaves. Drizzle with olive oil. Season with sea salt and pepper.

Nutrition Facts Per Serving:

310.6 calories; 17.9 g protein; 6.6 g carbohydrates; 59.8 mg cholesterol; 627.3 mg sodium.

Grilled Asparagus

Ingredients

1 pound fresh asparagus spears, trimmed

1 tablespoon olive oil

salt and pepper to taste

Directions

Step 1

Preheat grill for high heat.

Step 2

Lightly coat the asparagus spears with olive oil. Season with salt and pepper to taste.

Step 3

Grill over high heat for 2 to 3 minutes, or to desired tenderness.

Nutrition Facts Per Serving:

53 calories; 3.5 g total fat; 0 mg cholesterol; 2 mg sodium. 4.4 g carbohydrates; 2.5 g protein

Easy Herb Roasted Turkey

Ingredients

1 (12 pound) whole turkey

¾ cup olive oil

2 tablespoons garlic powder

2 teaspoons dried basil

1 teaspoon ground sage

1 teaspoon salt

½ teaspoon black pepper

2 cups water

Directions

Step 1

Preheat oven to 325 degrees F (165 degrees C). Clean turkey (discard giblets and organs), and place in a roasting pan with a lid.

Step 2

In a small bowl, combine olive oil, garlic powder, dried basil, ground sage, salt, and black pepper. Using a basting brush, apply the mixture to the outside of the uncooked turkey. Pour water into the bottom of the roasting pan, and cover.

Step 3

Bake for 3 to 3 1/2 hours, or until the internal temperature of the thickest part of the thigh measures 180 degrees F (82 degrees C). Remove bird from oven, and allow to stand for about 30 minutes before carving.

Nutrition Facts Per Serving:

596.8 calories; 68.2 g protein; 0.9 g carbohydrates; 198.3 mg cholesterol; 311.3 mg sodium.

Best Marinara Sauce Yet

Ingredient

2 (14.5 ounce) cans stewed tomatoes

1 (6 ounce) can tomato paste

4 tablespoons chopped fresh parsley

1 clove garlic, minced

1 teaspoon dried oregano

1 teaspoon salt

¼ teaspoon ground black pepper

6 tablespoons olive oil

⅓ cup finely diced onion

½ cup white wine

Directions

Step 1

In a food processor place Italian tomatoes, tomato paste, chopped parsley, minced garlic, oregano, salt, and pepper. Blend until smooth.

Step 2

In a large skillet over medium heat saute the finely chopped onion in olive oil for 2 minutes. Add the blended tomato sauce and white wine.

Step 3

Simmer for 30 minutes, stirring occasionally.

Nutrition Facts Per Serving:

150.8 calories; 2 g protein; 11.7 g carbohydrates; 0 mg cholesterol; 685.3 mg sodium.

Spaghetti Sauce with Ground Beef

Ingredients

1 pound ground beef

1 onion, chopped

4 cloves garlic, minced

1 small green bell pepper, diced

1 (28 ounce) can diced tomatoes

1 (16 ounce) can tomato sauce

1 (6 ounce) can tomato paste

2 teaspoons dried oregano

2 teaspoons dried basil

1 teaspoon salt

½ teaspoon black pepper

Directions

Step 1

Combine ground beef, onion, garlic, and green pepper in a large saucepan. Cook and stir until meat is brown and vegetables are tender. Drain grease.

Step 2

Stir diced tomatoes, tomato sauce, and tomato paste into the pan. Season with oregano, basil, salt, and pepper. Simmer spaghetti sauce for 1 hour, stirring occasionally.

Nutrition Facts Per Serving:

185.1 calories; 12.4 g protein; 15 g carbohydrates; 34.8 mg cholesterol; 930.8 mg sodium.

Homemade Taco Seasoning Mix

Ingredients

2 teaspoons hot chili powder

1 ½ teaspoons paprika

1 teaspoon onion powder

½ teaspoon sea salt

½ teaspoon garlic powder

½ teaspoon ground cumin

½ teaspoon oregano

¼ teaspoon freshly ground black pepper, or to taste

1 pinch cayenne pepper, or to taste

1 pinch red pepper flakes, or to taste

Directions

Step 1

Mix chili powder, paprika, onion powder, sea salt, garlic powder, cumin, oregano, black pepper, cayenne pepper, and red pepper flakes in a bowl.

Nutrition Facts Per Serving:

12.4 calories; 0.5 g protein; 2.4 g carbohydrates; 0 mg cholesterol; 234.7 mg sodium.

Roasted Okra

Ingredients

18 eaches fresh okra pods, sliced 1/3 inch thick

1 tablespoon olive oil

2 teaspoons kosher salt, or to taste

2 teaspoons black pepper, or to taste

Directions

Step 1

Preheat an oven to 425 degrees F (220 degrees C).

Step 2

Arrange the okra slices in one layer on a foil lined cookie sheet. Drizzle with olive oil and sprinkle with salt and pepper. Bake in the preheated oven for 10 to 15 minutes.

Nutrition Facts Per Serving:

65.4 calories; 1.6 g protein; 5.9 g carbohydrates; 0 mg cholesterol; 1286.4 mg sodium.

Roasted Asparagus Prosciutto and Egg

Ingredients

1 bunch fresh asparagus, trimmed

1 tablespoon extra-virgin olive oil

1 tablespoon olive oil

2 ounces minced prosciutto

ground black pepper

1 teaspoon distilled white vinegar

1 pinch salt

4 eggs

½ lemon, zested and juiced

1 pinch ground black pepper

Directions

Step 1

Preheat oven to 425 degrees F (220 degrees C). Place asparagus in a baking dish and drizzle with 1 tablespoon extra-virgin olive oil.

Step 2

Heat 1 tablespoon olive oil in a skillet over medium-low heat. Add prosciutto; cook, stirring, until golden and rendered, 3 to 4 minutes. Sprinkle prosciutto and oil over asparagus. Season with black pepper and toss to coat. Roast in the preheated oven for 10 minutes. Toss and return to oven until firm yet tender to the bite, 5 minutes.

Step 3

Fill a large saucepan with 2 to 3 inches of water and bring to a boil over high heat. Reduce heat to medium-low, pour in vinegar and pinch of salt. Crack an egg into a bowl then gently slip the egg into the water. Repeat with remaining eggs. Poach eggs until whites are firm and yolks have thickened but are not hard, 4 to 6 minutes. Remove eggs from water with a slotted spoon, dab on a kitchen towel to remove excess water, then transfer to a warm plate.

Step 4

Drizzle asparagus with lemon juice. Transfer asparagus to plates, top with poached egg and pinch of lemon zest. Season with black pepper and serve.

Nutrition Facts Per Serving:

199 calories; 15.7 g total fat; 175 mg cholesterol; 446 mg sodium. 5.1 g carbohydrates; 10.8 g protein

Ken's Perfect Hard Boiled Egg

Ingredient

1 tablespoon salt

¼ cup distilled white vinegar

6 cups water

8 eggs

Directions

Step 1

Combine the salt, vinegar, and water in a large pot, and bring to a boil over high heat. Add the eggs one at a time, being careful not to crack them. Reduce the heat to a gentle boil, and cook for 14 minutes.

Step 2

Once the eggs have cooked, remove them from the hot water, and place into a container of ice water or cold, running water. Cool completely, about 15 minutes. Store in the refrigerator up to 1 week.

Nutrition Facts Per Serving:

71.7 calories; 6.3 g protein; 0. 4 g carbohydrates; 186 mg cholesterol; 947.4 mg sodium.

Spicy Garlic Lime Chicken

Ingredients

3/4 teaspoon salt

1/4 teaspoon black pepper

1/4 teaspoon cayenne pepper

1/8 teaspoon paprika

1/4 teaspoon garlic powder

1/8 teaspoon onion powder

1/4 teaspoon dried thyme

1/4 teaspoon dried parsley

4 boneless, skinless chicken breast halves

2 tablespoons butter

1 tablespoon olive oil

2 teaspoons garlic powder

3 tablespoons lime juice

Directions

In a small bowl, mix together salt, black pepper, cayenne, paprika, 1/4 teaspoon garlic powder, onion powder, thyme and parsley. Sprinkle spice mixture generously on both sides of chicken breasts.

Heat butter and olive oil in a large heavy skillet over medium heat. Saute chicken until golden brown, about 6 minutes on each side. Sprinkle with 2 teaspoons garlic powder and lime juice. Cook 5 minutes more, stirring frequently to coat evenly with sauce.

Nutrition Facts Per Serving:

220 calories; 10.7 g fat; 2.4 g carbohydrates; 27.7 g protein; 84 mg cholesterol; 555 mg sodium. Full nutrition

Sweet, Sticky and Spicy Chicken

Ingredients

1 tablespoon brown sugar

2 tablespoons honey

¼ cup soy sauce

2 teaspoons chopped fresh ginger root

2 teaspoons chopped garlic

2 tablespoons hot sauce

1 pinch salt and pepper to taste

4 breast half, bone and skin removed (blank)s skinless, boneless chicken breast halves - cut into 1/2 inch strips

1 tablespoon vegetable oil

Directions

Step 1

Mix together brown sugar, honey, soy sauce, ginger, garlic and hot sauce in a small bowl.

Step 2

Lightly salt and pepper the chicken strips.

Step 3

Heat oil in a large skillet over medium heat. Add chicken strips and brown on both sides, about 1 minute per side. Pour the sauce over the chicken. Simmer uncovered until the sauce thickens, 8 to 10 minutes.

Nutrition Facts Per Serving:

232.4 calories; 22.8 g protein; 13.9 g carbohydrates; 59.3 mg cholesterol; 1176.2 mg sodium.

Chicken Breasts in Caper Cream Sauce

Ingredients

4 breast half, bone and skin removed (blank)s boneless, skinless chicken breast halves

1 teaspoon lemon pepper

1 teaspoon salt

1 teaspoon dried dill weed

1 teaspoon garlic powder

3 tablespoons butter

½ cup whipping cream

2 tablespoons capers, drained and rinsed

Directions

Step 1

Season chicken breasts with lemon pepper, salt, dill weed, and garlic powder.

Step 2

Melt butter in a large skillet over medium heat. Place breasts in skillet, and increase heat to medium-high. Turn chicken frequently, until brown, about 5 minutes. Reduce heat to medium, and cook 5 to 7 minutes, until breasts are cooked through. Remove chicken to a warm serving platter, and cover with foil.

Step 3

Return skillet to stove, and increase heat to high. Whisk in whipping cream, whisking continuously until reduced to sauce consistency, about 3 minutes. Remove from heat. Stir in capers. Pour sauce over chicken, and serve.

Nutrition Facts Per Serving:

313.3 calories; 28.2 g protein; 1.8 g carbohydrates; 132.1 mg cholesterol; 974.3 mg sodium.

Dijon-Tarragon Cream Chicken

Ingredients

1 tablespoon butter

1 tablespoon olive oil

4 breast half, bone and skin removed (blank)s skinless, boneless chicken breast halves

1 pinch salt and pepper to taste

½ cup heavy cream

1 tablespoon Dijon mustard

2 teaspoons chopped fresh tarragon

Directions

Step 1

Melt the butter and heat the oil in a skillet over medium-high heat. Season chicken with salt and pepper, and place in the skillet. Brown on both sides. Reduce heat to medium, cover, and continue cooking 15 minutes, or until chicken juices run clear. Set aside and keep warm.

Step 2

Stir cream into the pan, scraping up brown bits. Mix in mustard and tarragon. Cook and stir 5 minutes, or until thickened. Return chicken to skillet to coat with sauce. Drizzle chicken with remaining sauce to serve.

Nutrition Facts Per Serving:

310.1 calories; 27.1 g protein; 2.1 g carbohydrates; 120.3 mg cholesterol; 226.8 mg sodium.

Sweet and Spicy Stir Fry with Chicken and Broccoli

Ingredients

3 cups broccoli florets

1 tablespoon olive oil

2 breast half, bone and skin removed (blank)s skinless, boneless chicken breast halves - cut into 1 inch strips

¼ cup sliced green onions

4 cloves garlic, thinly sliced

1 tablespoon hoisin sauce

1 tablespoon chile paste

1 tablespoon low sodium soy sauce

½ teaspoon ground ginger

¼ teaspoon crushed red pepper

½ teaspoon salt

½ teaspoon black pepper

⅛ cup chicken stock

Directions

Step 1

Place broccoli in a steamer over 1 inch of boiling water, and cover. Cook until tender but still firm, about 5 minutes.

Step 2

Heat the oil in a skillet over medium heat, and saute the chicken, green onions, and garlic until the chicken is no longer pink and juices run clear.

Step 3

Stir the hoisin sauce, chile paste, and soy sauce into the skillet; season with ginger, red pepper, salt, and black pepper. Stir in the chicken stock and simmer about 2 minutes. Mix in the steamed broccoli until coated with the sauce mixture.

Nutrition Facts Per Serving:

155.9 calories; 15.9 g protein; 10.9 g carbohydrates; 36.2 mg cholesterol; 606.4 mg sodium.

Perfect Turkey
Ingredients

1 (18 pound) whole turkey, neck and giblets removed

2 cups kosher salt

1/2 cup butter, melted

2 large onions, peeled and chopped

4 carrots, peeled and chopped

4 stalks celery, chopped

2 sprigs fresh thyme

1 bay leaf

1 cup dry white wine

Directions

Rub the turkey inside and out with the kosher salt. Place the bird in a large stock pot, and cover with cold water. Place in the refrigerator, and allow the turkey to soak in the salt and water mixture 12 hours, or overnight.

Preheat oven to 350 degrees F (175 degrees C). Thoroughly rinse the turkey, and discard the brine mixture.

Brush the turkey with 1/2 the melted butter. Place breast side down on a roasting rack in a shallow roasting pan. Stuff the turkey cavity with 1 onion, 1/2 the carrots, 1/2 the celery, 1 sprig of thyme, and the bay leaf. Scatter the remaining vegetables and thyme around the bottom of the roasting pan, and cover with the white wine.

Roast uncovered 3 1/2 to 4 hours in the preheated oven, until the internal temperature of the thigh reaches 180 degrees F (85 degrees C). Carefully turn the turkey breast side up about 2/3 through the roasting time, and brush with the remaining butter. Allow the bird to stand about 30 minutes before carving.

Crispy Rosemary Chicken and Fries

Ingredients

8 thigh, bone removeds chicken thighs

6 small red potatoes, quartered

½ cup extra-virgin olive oil, or as needed

1 tablespoon chopped fresh rosemary

1 ½ teaspoons chopped fresh oregano

1 ½ teaspoons garlic powder

1 pinch salt and pepper to taste

Directions

Step 1

Preheat the oven to 375 degrees F (190 degrees C).

Step 2

Place chicken and potatoes into a large bowl. Pour olive oil over them, and stir to coat. Scatter the chicken and potato pieces in a large baking dish, or cookie sheet with sides. Sprinkle with rosemary, oregano, garlic powder, salt and pepper.

Step 3

Bake for 1 hour in the preheated oven, uncovered. Baste during the last 15 minutes for extra crispness.

Nutrition Facts Per Serving:

497.1 calories; 24.4 g protein; 27.6 g carbohydrates; 78 mg cholesterol; 106.7 mg sodium.

Chef John's Make-Ahead Turkey Gravy

Ingredients

1 large onion, chopped

2 carrots, chopped

2 ribs celery, chopped

2 teaspoons vegetable oil

2 large turkey wings

2 tablespoons cold water

10 cups cold water

4 sprigs fresh thyme

2 cloves garlic (optional)

3 tablespoons butter

1/2 cup all-purpose flour

salt and ground black pepper to taste

1 pinch cayenne pepper

Directions

Preheat oven to 400 degrees F (200 degrees C).

Combine onion, carrots, celery, and vegetable oil in a large roasting pan and toss to coat. Place turkey wings on top of vegetables

Place roasting pan in the preheated oven and cook until the turkey wings are browned and vegetables are caramelized and softened, 45 to 60 minutes.

Transfer turkey wings and vegetables to a large stockpot. Place the roasting pan over a stovetop burner on medium heat. Pour 2 tablespoons cold water into the pan and bring to a boil, scraping up any browned bits. Transfer mixture to the stockpot and add 10 cups cold water, thyme, and garlic.

Bring turkey wing mixture to a boil. Reduce heat to low and simmer, uncovered, until meat falls off the bone, about 3 hours. Skim off turkey fat throughout the process and set aside 2 tablespoons.

Strain turkey stock and reserve 6 cups of stock; discard all the solids.

Heat butter and 2 tablespoons reserved turkey fat in a large saucepan over medium heat. Sprinkle in flour and cook, whisking continuously, until it begins to smell like cooked pie crust, 2 to 3 minutes. Slowly pour in turkey stock, whisking continuously. Increase heat to high and simmer until thick and warmed through, about 5 minutes. Season with salt, black pepper, and cayenne pepper to taste.

Nutrition Facts Per Serving:

115 calories; 6.6 g fat; 10.2 g carbohydrates; 4.1 g protein; 23 mg cholesterol; 92 mg sodium.

Suki's Spinach and Feta Pasta

Ingredients

1 (8 ounce) package penne pasta

2 tablespoons olive oil

1/2 cup chopped onion

1 clove garlic, minced

3 cups chopped tomatoes

1 cup sliced fresh mushrooms

2 cups spinach leaves, packed

salt and pepper to taste

1 pinch red pepper flakes

8 ounces feta cheese, crumbled

Directions

Bring a large pot of lightly salted water to a boil. Cook pasta in boiling water until al dente; drain.

Meanwhile, heat olive oil in a large skillet over medium-high heat; add onion and garlic, and cook until golden brown. Mix in tomatoes, mushrooms, and spinach. Season with salt, pepper, and red pepper flakes. Cook 2 minutes more, until tomatoes are heated through and spinach is wilted. Reduce heat to medium, stir in pasta and feta cheese, and cook until heated through.

Aunt Carol's Spinach and Fish Bake

Ingredients

1 (10 ounce) package frozen chopped spinach, thawed and squeezed dry

1 cup sharp Cheddar cheese

1/3 cup dry bread crumbs

1 egg, beaten

1 pound cod fillets

salt and pepper to taste

Directions

Preheat oven to 325 degrees F (165 degrees C).

In a bowl, mix the spinach, 1/2 cup Cheddar cheese, about 5 tablespoons dry bread crumbs, and the egg. Spread the mixture into the bottom of a small baking dish.

Arrange the cod fillets on top of the spinach mixture, and season with salt and pepper. Top with the remaining Cheddar cheese and bread crumbs.

Cover, and bake 20 minutes in the preheated oven, or until fish flakes easily with a fork.

Nutrition Facts Per Serving:

306 calories; 14.3 g fat; 10 g carbohydrates; 34.2 g protein; 131 mg cholesterol; 419 mg sodium.

Perfect Ten Baked Cod

Ingredients

2 tablespoons butter

1/2 sleeve buttery round crackers (such as Ritz®), crushed

2 tablespoons butter

1 pound thick-cut cod loin

1/2 lemon, juiced

1/4 cup dry white wine

1 tablespoon chopped fresh parsley

1 tablespoon chopped green onion

1 lemon, cut into wedges

Directions

Preheat oven to 400 degrees F (200 degrees C).

Place 2 tablespoons butter in a microwave-safe bowl; melt in microwave on high, about 30 seconds. Stir buttery round crackers into melted butter.

Place remaining 2 tablespoons butter in a 7x11-inch baking dish. Melt in the preheated oven, 1 to 3 minutes. Remove dish from oven.

Coat both sides of cod in melted butter in the baking dish.

Bake cod in the preheated oven for 10 minutes. Remove from oven; top with lemon juice, wine, and cracker mixture. Place back in oven and bake until fish is opaque and flakes easily with a fork, about 10 more minutes.

Garnish baked cod with parsley and green onion. Serve with lemon wedges.

Nutrition Facts Per Serving: 280 calories; 16.1 g fat; 9.3 g carbohydrates; 20.9 g protein; 71 mg cholesterol; 282 mg sodium.

Baked Salmon Fillets Dijon

Ingredients

4 (4 ounce) fillets salmon

3 tablespoons prepared Dijon-style mustard

salt and pepper to taste

1/4 cup Italian-style dry bread crumbs

1/4 cup butter, melted

Directions

Preheat oven to 400 degrees F (200 degrees C). Line a shallow baking pan with aluminum foil.

Place salmon skin-side down on foil. Spread a thin layer of mustard on the top of each fillet, and season with salt and pepper. Top with bread crumbs, then drizzle with melted butter.

Bake in a preheated oven for 15 minutes, or until salmon flakes easily with a fork.

Nutrition Facts Per Serving:

331 calories; 21.5 g fat; 7.5 g carbohydrates; 25 g protein; 106 mg cholesterol; 552 mg sodium.

Baked Lemon Chicken with Mushroom Sauce

Ingredients

1 tablespoon olive oil

6 skinless, boneless chicken breast halves

1 lemon

1/4 cup butter

3 cups fresh sliced mushrooms

2 tablespoons all-purpose flour

1/2 cup chicken broth, or more as needed

1 tablespoon chopped fresh parsley

Directions

Preheat oven to 400 degrees F (205 degrees C).

Pour olive oil in an 8x8-inch glass baking dish. Place the chicken breasts in the dish, coating each side with oil. Squeeze the juice of 1/2 lemon over each chicken breast. Slice the rest of the lemon and place a lemon slice on top of each chicken piece.

Bake in the preheated oven until no longer pink in the center and the juices run clear, 30 to 40 minutes. An instant-read thermometer inserted into the center should read at least 165 degrees F (74 degrees C).

Melt butter in a skillet over medium heat; add mushrooms. Cook and stir until mushrooms are brown and liquid is evaporated, about 6 minutes. Sprinkle flour over mushrooms and stir until coated. Add chicken broth, stirring to make a medium-thick sauce. Allow sauce to reduce, adjusting with a little more broth to make a creamy sauce. Add fresh parsley at the last minute. Spoon the sauce over the baked chicken breasts.

Nutrition Facts Per Serving:

240 calories; 13 g fat; 5.2 g carbohydrates; 26.3 g protein; 88 mg cholesterol; 196 mg sodium.

Curried Honey Mustard Chicken

Ingredients

1/3 cup butter, melted

1/3 cup honey

1/4 cup Dijon-style prepared mustard

4 teaspoons curry powder

1 pinch ground cayenne pepper

4 skinless, boneless chicken breasts

Directions

In a medium bowl combine the melted butter/margarine, honey, mustard, curry powder and cayenne powder. Mix well. Place chicken breasts in a 9x13 inch baking dish and pour honey/mustard mixture over chicken. Cover and place in refrigerator. Marinate for at least 4 hours or overnight.

Preheat oven to 375 degrees F (190 degrees C).

Remove dish from refrigerator and bake, covered, in the preheated oven for 10 minutes. Remove cover and bake about 10 minutes more, or until done and juices run clear (baking time will depend a little on how thick your chicken breasts are).

Nutrition Facts Per Serving:

 374 calories; 17.1 g fat; 27.6 g carbohydrates; 27.8 g protein; 109 mg cholesterol; 563 mg sodium.

Butternut Squash Soup II

Ingredients

2 tablespoons butter

1 small onion, chopped

1 stalk celery, chopped

1 medium carrot, chopped

2 medium potatoes, cubed

1 medium butternut squash - peeled, seeded, and cubed

1 (32 fluid ounce) container chicken stock

salt and freshly ground black pepper to taste

Directions

Melt the butter in a large pot, and cook the onion, celery, carrot, potatoes, and squash 5 minutes, or until lightly browned. Pour in enough of the chicken stock to cover vegetables. Bring to a boil. Reduce heat to low, cover pot, and simmer 40 minutes, or until all vegetables are tender.

Transfer the soup to a blender, and blend until smooth. Return to pot, and mix in any remaining stock to attain desired consistency. Season with salt and pepper.

Nutrition Facts Per Serving:

 305 calories; 6.8 g fat; 59.7 g carbohydrates; 6.9 g protein; 21 mg cholesterol; 1151 mg sodium.

Butternut Squash Bisque

Ingredients

1 tablespoon canola oil

1 tablespoon unsalted butter

1/2 cup diced onion

3/4 cup diced carrots

4 cups peeled and cubed butternut squash

3 cups vegetable stock

salt and ground black pepper to taste

ground nutmeg to taste

1/2 cup heavy cream (optional)

Add all ingredients to list

Directions

Heat the oil and melt the butter in a large pot over medium heat. Cook and stir the onion in the butter and oil under tender.

Mix the carrots and squash into the pot. Pour in vegetable stock, and season with salt, pepper, and nutmeg. Bring to a boil, reduce heat, and simmer until vegetables are tender.

In a blender or food processor, puree the soup mixture until smooth. Return to the pot, and stir in the heavy cream. Heat through, but do not boil. Serve warm with a dash of nutmeg.

Nutrition Facts Per Serving:

 248 calories; 18.2 g fat; 21.8 g carbohydrates; 2.7 g protein; 48 mg cholesterol; 820 mg sodium.

Butternut Squash and Turkey Chili
Ingredients

2 tablespoons olive oil

1 onion, chopped

2 cloves garlic, minced

1 pound ground turkey breast

1 pound butternut squash - peeled, seeded and cut into 1-inch dice

½ cup chicken broth

1 (4.5 ounce) can chopped green chilies

2 (14.5 ounce) cans petite diced tomatoes

1 (15 ounce) can kidney beans with liquid

1 (15.5 ounce) can white hominy, drained

1 (8 ounce) can tomato sauce

1 tablespoon chili powder

1 tablespoon ground cumin

1 teaspoon garlic salt

Directions

Step 1

Heat the olive oil in a large pot over medium heat. Stir in the onion and garlic; cook and stir for 3 minutes, then add the turkey, and stir until crumbly and no longer pink.

Step 2

Add the butternut squash, chicken broth, green chilies, tomatoes, kidney beans, hominy, and tomato sauce; season with chili powder, cumin, and garlic salt. Bring to a simmer, then reduce heat to medium-low, cover, and simmer until the squash is tender, about 20 minutes.

Nutrition Facts Per Serving:

165 calories; 13.4 g protein; 20.5 g carbohydrates; 23.7 mg cholesterol; 709.2 mg sodium. Full Nutrition

Butternut Squash Pizzas with Rosemary

Ingredients

1 cup thinly sliced onion

1/2 butternut squash - peeled, seeded, and thinly sliced

1 teaspoon chopped fresh rosemary

salt and black pepper to taste

3 tablespoons olive oil, divided

1 (16 ounce) package refrigerated pizza crust dough, divided

1 tablespoon cornmeal

2 tablespoons grated Asiago or Parmesan cheese

Directions

Preheat oven to 400 degrees F (205 degrees C). Place sliced onion and squash in a roasting pan. Sprinkle with rosemary, salt, pepper, and 2 tablespoons of the olive oil; toss to coat.

Bake in the preheated oven for 20 minutes, or until onions are lightly browned and squash is tender; set aside.

Increase oven temperature to 450 degrees F (230 degrees C). On a floured surface, roll each ball of dough into an 8 inch round. Place the rounds on a baking sheet sprinkled with cornmeal (you may need 2 baking sheets depending on their size). Distribute squash mixture over the two rounds and continue baking for 10 minutes, checking occasionally, or until the crust is firm. Sprinkle with cheese and remaining tablespoon olive oil. Cut into quarters, and serve.

Nutrition Facts Per Serving:

 567 calories; 13.7 g fat; 96.9 g carbohydrates; 14.8 g protein; 3 mg cholesterol; 948 mg sodium.

Roasted Butternut Squash and Garlic Lasagna

Ingredients

3 pounds butternut squash, halved and seeded

3 tablespoons vegetable oil

1/2 teaspoon salt

1/4 cup unsalted butter

2 tablespoons minced garlic

1/4 cup all-purpose flour

1 quart milk

salt and ground black pepper to taste

1 cup heavy cream

9 no-cook lasagna noodles

1 1/3 cups finely grated Parmesan cheese

Directions

Preheat an oven to 450 degrees F (230 degrees C). Grease a baking sheet.

Brush the butternut squash halves with vegetable oil and season with salt. Roast in the preheated oven until golden and easily pierced with a knife, 45 to 50 minutes. Allow to cool for 15 to 20 minutes, then scoop the flesh into a bowl. Set aside.

Heat the butter in a large skillet over medium-low heat. Cook and stir garlic in the butter until softened. Stir in flour and cook for 3 minutes. Whisk in the milk until smooth. Bring to a simmer, and cook until thick, about 10 minutes, whisking occasionally. Stir in the butternut squash and season with salt and pepper. Sauce can be made 3 days ahead and refrigerated.

Reduce oven temperature to to 375 degrees F (190 degrees C). Grease a 9x13 inch baking dish.

Beat the heavy cream until foamy in a large glass or metal mixing bowl. Gradually add the salt, continuing to beat until medium peaks form. Lift your beater or whisk straight up: the tip of the peak formed by the cream should curl over slightly. Set aside.

Pour 1 cup of the butternut sauce into the baking dish and place 3 lasagna noodles on top in a single layer. Spread half of the remaining sauce over the noodles and sprinkle with 1/2 cup of Parmesan cheese. Place another layer of noodles and spread the remaining sauce on top and sprinkle with 1/2 cup of Parmesan cheese. Place the final layer of noodles on top. Spread the whipped cream over the final layer of noodles making sure the pasta is completely covered. Sprinkle with the remaining 1/3 cup of Parmesan. Cover baking dish tightly with aluminum foil.

Bake in the preheated oven for 30 minutes. Remove foil and continue baking until the top is bubbly and golden brown, about 10 minutes. Allow to rest for 5 minutes before serving.

Nutrition Facts Per Serving:

339 calories; 19.3 g fat; 33.5 g carbohydrates; 10.4 g protein; 52 mg cholesterol; 293 mg sodium.

Roasted Asparagus with Parmesan

Ingredients

olive oil cooking spray

1 pound fresh asparagus, tough ends trimmed

1/4 cup shredded Parmesan cheese

1 teaspoon sea salt

1/4 teaspoon garlic powder, or to taste

Directions

Preheat oven to 400 degrees F (200 degrees C).

Spray the inside of a 9x13 casserole dish with olive oil cooking spray. Place asparagus in the dish and lightly spray spears with cooking spray.

Sprinkle asparagus with Parmesan cheese, sea salt, and garlic powder.

Roast in preheated oven until fork easily punctures thickest part of stem, about 12 minutes.

Nutrition Facts Per Serving: 46 calories;

1.7 g fat; 4.7 g carbohydrates; 4.4 g protein; 4 mg cholesterol; 660 mg sodium.

Grilled Garlic Parmesan Zucchini

Ingredients

3 zucchini

3 tablespoons butter, softened

2 cloves garlic, minced

1 tablespoon chopped fresh parsley

1/2 cup freshly grated Parmesan cheese

Add all ingredients to list

Directions

Preheat an outdoor grill for medium-high heat, and lightly oil the grate.

Cut the zucchini in half crosswise, then slice each half into 3 slices lengthwise, making 6 slices per zucchini.

Mix the butter, garlic, and parsley in a bowl, and spread the mixture on both sides of each zucchini slice. Sprinkle one side of each slice with Parmesan cheese, and place the slices, cheese sides up, crosswise on the preheated grill to keep them from falling through.

Grill the zucchini until the cheese has melted and the slices are cooked through and show grill marks, about 8 minutes.

Nutrition Facts Per Serving:

146 calories; 11.8 g fat; 5.9 g carbohydrates; 5.8 g protein; 32 mg cholesterol; 230 mg sodium.

Spicy Bok Choy in Garlic Sauce

Ingredients

1 pound bok choy

1 tablespoon vegetable oil

1 tablespoon sesame oil

1/4 cup water

1 teaspoon grated fresh ginger root

2 cloves garlic, minced

1 tablespoon oyster sauce

1 tablespoon light soy sauce

1 tablespoon brown sugar

1/8 teaspoon crushed red pepper flakes (optional)

Directions

Trim off the ends of the bok choy and chop, keeping the white parts separate from the green as they will need to cook longer. Rinse and spin or pat dry. Set aside.

In a small bowl or cup, stir together the vegetable oil and sesame oil. In a separate larger bowl, stir together the water, ginger, garlic, oyster sauce, soy sauce, brown sugar and red pepper flakes. Set this aside.

Heat the oil in a large skillet or wok over medium-high heat. Add the bok choy stems first; stir fry for a few minutes or until the pieces start to turn a pale green. When stems are almost cooked, add the leaves; cook and stir until leaves are wilted, 1 to 2 minutes. Remove from the heat and transfer the bok choy to a serving dish. Pour the sauce into the skillet or wok, and set over medium-high heat. Cook, stirring constantly, until sauce has thickened slightly, about 3 minutes. Pour over the bok choy and toss lightly to coat.

Nutrition Facts Per Serving:

93 calories; 7.1 g fat; 6.9 g carbohydrates; 2 g protein; 0 mg cholesterol; 236 mg sodium.

Garlic Mashed Cauliflower

Ingredients

1 head cauliflower, cut into florets

1 tablespoon olive oil

1 clove garlic, smashed

1/4 cup grated Parmesan cheese

1 tablespoon reduced-fat cream cheese

1/2 teaspoon kosher salt

1/8 teaspoon freshly ground black pepper

Directions

Place a steamer insert into a saucepan and fill with water to just below the bottom of the steamer. Bring water to a boil. Add cauliflower, cover, and steam until tender, about 10 minutes.

Meanwhile, heat olive oil in a small skillet over medium heat; cook and stir garlic until softened, about 2 minutes. Remove from heat.

Transfer half the cauliflower to a food processor; cover and blend on high. Add remaining cauliflower florets, one at a time, until vegetables are creamy. Blend in garlic, Parmesan cheese, cream cheese, salt, and black pepper.

Nutrition Facts Per Serving:

98 calories; 5.7 g fat; 8.4 g carbohydrates; 5.2 g protein; 7 mg cholesterol; 372 mg sodium.

Roasted Balsamic Cauliflower

Ingredients

2 tablespoons olive oil

2 tablespoons balsamic vinegar

1/2 teaspoon salt

3 cloves garlic, chopped

1 head cauliflower, chopped into bite size pieces

Directions

Preheat oven to 450 degrees F (230 degrees C). Line a baking sheet with aluminum foil

Stir the olive oil, balsamic vinegar, salt, and garlic together in a bowl. Add the cauliflower and toss to coat; spread the mixture onto the lined baking sheet.

Stirring occasionally, bake in the preheated oven until tender, about 20 minutes.

Nutrition Facts Per Serving:

86 calories; 5.7 g fat; 7.7 g carbohydrates; 3.1 g protein; 0 mg cholesterol; 257 mg sodium.